NAVIGATING GIANT CELL TUMOR OF BONE WITH CONFIDENCE AND CARE

Empowering Strategies And Unveiling The Path For Quick Approach To Bone Healing For Healthy Relief

DR. WESLEY IAN

DISCLAIMER

The information in this book is not meant to replace professional medical advice, diagnosis, or treatment; rather, it is meant mainly for general informational reasons. If you have any questions about a medical problem, you should always consult your doctor or another trained health expert. Don't ever discount expert medical advice or put off getting it because of something you've read in this book.

Any negative effects or repercussions arising from the usage of the material provided herein are not the responsibility of the book's author or publisher. It should be noted by readers that the material in this book is not all-inclusive and might not address every facet of the subject. Furthermore, new research may have an impact on how health concerns are understood or treated because medical knowledge is always changing.

No particular test, treatment, method, or product mentioned in this book is endorsed or promoted by the author or publisher. The reader assumes all risk associated with using the information included in this book.

Before making any big decisions regarding your health, it's crucial to speak with a licensed healthcare provider. The relationship between a patient and their healthcare practitioner should not be replaced by this book, nor is it meant to offer medical advice.

The opinions presented in this book are the author's and may not necessarily represent those of the publisher. Any errors, omissions, or inaccuracies in the information in this book are not the responsibility of the author or publisher.

It is recommended that readers independently confirm any information contained in this book and speak with a healthcare provider about their specific medical needs and state of health.

TABLE OF CONTENTS

ABOUT THE BOOK

In the field of medical literature, "Navigating Giant Cell Tumor of Bone with Confidence and Care" is an excellent resource that offers a thorough manual for both patients and medical professionals. The book is organized to provide readers with a comprehensive grasp of the complications surrounding giant cell tumors. It includes insights into diagnosis, medical management, holistic care, patient views, navigating the healthcare system, and life following treatment.

The backdrop and overview of giant cell tumors, the book's goal, and the intended readership are all provided in the opening section, which also establishes the scene. The reader's engagement is established by this contextualization, which also emphasizes the significance of the material that follows.

"Understanding Giant Cell Tumor of Bone," the second segment, explores the fundamental features of the illness. This section offers a comprehensive investigation of the condition, from its definition and characteristics to its causes, risk factors, typical locations in the body, and indications and symptoms, ensuring readers get a strong understanding of it.

The book then smoothly moves into the diagnostic stage, explaining the importance of the patient's medical history, physical examination, imaging methods, biopsy procedures, and laboratory testing. Through the illumination of these crucial components, the book equips medical professionals and patients with the necessary knowledge to make prompt and correct diagnoses.

The fourth section is devoted to the medical treatment of giant cell tumors. Conventional treatment modalities, such as radiation therapy and surgery, are very specific. Furthermore, a comprehensive understanding of the treatment environment is provided by investigating new treatments and innovations as well as providing insights into possible side effects and complications. Additionally, the section offers advice on how to get ready for these therapies so that people can make well-informed decisions.

The fifth segment emphasizes the connection between physical and emotional well-being by discussing integrative medicine, diet, lifestyle factors, and pain treatment. It does this by acknowledging the significance of a holistic approach to care. The sixth section's patient perspectives and anecdotes add a human touch to the medical material previously offered by sharing real-life experiences and coping mechanisms.

The seventh portion covers managing the healthcare system, including how to assemble a healthcare team, communicate with specialists effectively, get second views, and comprehend financial and insurance implications. This section acts as a helpful manual to help readers take an active role in their healthcare journey.

The eighth and last section discusses life after treatment, covering topics such as follow-up care, long-term monitoring, survivorship, healing, rehabilitation, and overcoming recurrence worry. This forward-thinking strategy guarantees that the book will continue to be a useful and encouraging resource for the duration of the healthcare process.

To put it simply, "Navigating Giant Cell Tumor of Bone with Confidence and Care" is a unique resource that goes beyond the scope of conventional medical literature. By combining medical expertise, patient stories, and helpful guidance, the book serves as a helpful guide for people navigating the complexities of giant cell tumors and emphasizes the value of making well-informed decisions and maintaining holistic well-being when dealing with a difficult medical condition.

CHAPTER ONE

INTRODUCTION TO GIANT CELL TUMOR OF BONE

NAVIGATING GIANT CELL TUMORS: AN IMPORTANT TASK

Because of the enormous consequences giant cell tumors (GCTs) have for the health of the musculoskeletal system, understanding their complexities is essential. Given that giant cell tumors are known to be locally aggressive and have the potential to recur, both patients and healthcare providers must comprehend and manage them well. Given the many side effects this tumor may cause, including bone loss, joint degeneration, and metastasis, it is critical to manage it.

A thorough investigation of this illness is necessary to guide treatment strategies, reduce related risks, and enhance patient outcomes.

COMPREHENDING BONE GIANT CELL TUMOR

A unique neoplasm, a giant cell tumor of the bone is identified by the presence of mononuclear, stromal, and multinucleated large cells. GCT is a benign, locally aggressive tumor, although it can be difficult to diagnose and cure. Its distinct identification within the spectrum of bone tumors is influenced by its histological characteristics, which include the presence of large cells within a neoplastic stromal background. Comprehending the subtleties of GCT histopathology is essential for a precise diagnosis, which opens the door to individualized treatment plans that complement the unique features of the tumor.

DEFINITION AND QUALITIES

The intricacy and variability of giant cell tumors are highlighted by their definition and characteristics. GCT arises from the bone stromal cells and presents a wide range of clinical characteristics. Some cases progress more slowly, while others become locally destructive lesions. Understanding the many ways in which this tumor presents itself is essential to creating customized treatment strategies that take into account the particulars of every patient.

Furthermore, the ability to foresee malignant change is essential for informing clinical judgment and guaranteeing prompt action when required.

REASONS AND DANGER ELEMENTS

Research and investigation into the causes and risk factors of giant cell tumors are continuing. Although the precise cause of GCT remains unclear, several variables, including age, gender, and genetic predisposition, have been linked to the condition. The multifactorial nature of GCT development is highlighted by a preference for people in their third and fourth decades of life, a little female predominance, and the possible impact of genetic alterations. Both focused therapy therapies and preventive measures require a comprehensive understanding of these relevant elements.

TYPICAL PLACES IN THE BODY

Big Cell Tumors frequently appear in the metaphyseal-epiphyseal region of long bones, especially in the area surrounding the knee joint. This preference for particular anatomical locations highlights the special milieu that supports the formation of GCT. Knowing the typical locations makes early detection and intervention easier, enabling medical professionals to adjust their treatment plans and diagnostic techniques appropriately. Furthermore, the preference for particular regions guides current investigations intended to elucidate the microenvironmental elements involved in the start and development of GCT.

SYMPTOMS AND INDICATIONS

Giant cell tumor symptoms and indicators cover a wide range of clinical manifestations, from moderate discomfort to excruciating pain and loss of function. People with GCT commonly experience localized discomfort, edema, and limited joint movement. It is essential to identify these clinical signs to enable prompt diagnosis and action. Moreover, the discovery of atypical presentations or asymptomatic instances highlights the necessity of an all-encompassing diagnostic strategy that takes into account radiological, histological, and clinical findings.

Understanding giant cell tumors requires a detailed investigation of their significance, definition, traits, origins, typical sites, and warning signs and symptoms. This complex knowledge is essential for researchers, doctors, and patients alike, as it serves as the basis for customized treatment plans, well-informed decision-making, and continuous progress in the field of musculoskeletal cancer.

CHAPTER TWO

A GIANT CELL TUMOR'S DIAGNOSIS

MEDICAL BACKGROUND AND PHYSICAL ASSESSMENT

The diagnosis of a giant cell tumor (GCT) begins with a complete medical history and physical examination. Information regarding the patient's symptoms, such as localized discomfort, edema, and restricted joint movement, is gathered by medical specialists. They also ask how long these symptoms have lasted and how they have progressed. The medical history also aids in determining any risk factors that may exist, such as prior trauma or underlying bone disorders.

Healthcare professionals evaluate the afflicted area during the physical examination, searching for indications of edema, discomfort, and variations in skin tone or temperature. They assess joint mobility and function as well. The basis for additional diagnostic research is laid by learning about the patient's medical history and doing a thorough physical examination.

IMAGING METHODS (MRIS, CT SCANS, AND X-RAYS)

Giant cell tumors are difficult to diagnose without imaging, which gives precise information about the tumor's location, size, and effects on adjacent structures. When it comes to identifying anomalies in bone structure, like regions of bone loss and the distinctive soap-bubble look associated with GCT, X-rays are frequently the first imaging modality to be used.

Magnesium Resonance Imaging, or MRI, is useful in determining the extent of soft tissue involvement and identifying alterations in bone marrow. It provides a closer look at the tumor and how it interacts with surrounding structures, which helps with surgical planning and assessing the disease's severity.

CT (Computerized Tomography) scans can be used to assess the bone lesions more thoroughly and provide more details about the tumor's features. This imaging method can supplement results from X-rays and MRIs and is especially helpful for evaluating the bone architecture.

METHODS FOR BIOPSIES

The process of removing a tiny sample of tissue for laboratory analysis, known as a biopsy, is frequently necessary to provide a conclusive diagnosis of a giant cell tumor. Numerous biopsy techniques exist, such as open biopsy and core needle biopsy. A core needle biopsy is a minimally invasive method in which a tissue sample is obtained by inserting a needle into the tumor. An open biopsy entails removing the tumor whole or in part surgically for analysis.

The biopsy helps rule out other bone disorders or cancers while confirming the existence of giant cell tumor cells. To identify hallmark signs of GCT, such as hemosiderin-laden macrophages, mononuclear stromal cells, and multinucleated giant cells, histopathological investigation of the biopsy sample is essential.

LABORATORY EXAMINATIONS

Even though laboratory tests cannot identify giant cell tumors directly, they can help rule out other illnesses and determine the patient's general state of health. To assess for any systemic abnormalities or underlying bone problems, blood tests may be conducted. These tests may include a complete blood count (CBC) and indicators of bone metabolism.

Increased bone turnover linked to giant cell tumors may be indicated by elevated levels of alkaline phosphatase and serum calcium. These markers, however, are not exclusive to GCT and can be raised in several different bone conditions. Laboratory testing is part of a comprehensive diagnostic approach for giant cell tumors, together with imaging and biopsy data.

CHAPTER THREE

MEDICAL HANDLING OF MASSIVE CELL TUMOR

CONVENTIONAL THERAPY METHODS

Usually affecting the metaphysis of long bones, giant cell tumors (GCTs) are an aggressive localized tumor that frequently affects young individuals. A multimodal strategy is used in the medical care of giant cell tumors, taking into account new and developing medicines as well as any possible side effects or problems.

Historically, the foundation of treatment for giant cell tumors has been surgery. The whole tumor removal with the function of the affected limb preserved is the main aim of surgery.

A popular surgical procedure called curettage involves scraping the tumor out of the bone; to aid in healing, bone grafting may come next. However, the possibility of recurrence still exists, especially when anatomical limitations make total removal impossible.

RADIATION TREATMENT

Another conventional therapeutic option for giant cell tumors is radiation therapy. It is frequently taken into consideration to lower the chance of recurrence following surgical intervention or when surgery is not practical. The goal of radiation therapy is to find and eliminate any remaining tumor cells. However, because of the possibility of long-term side effects such as radiation-induced sarcomas and poor bone repair, it is not the first-line treatment.

NEW TREATMENTS AND DEVELOPMENTS

Recent years have seen promise in the development of novel treatments and improvements in the medical care of giant cell tumors. Tumor growth and symptoms have been effectively reduced by denosumab, a monoclonal antibody that inhibits the receptor activator of nuclear factor-kappa B ligand (RANKL). For patients who might not be good candidates for conventional procedures, this tailored therapy has given them a non-surgical alternative.

ADVERSE REACTIONS AND ISSUES

The treatment modalities selected for Giant Cell Tumors can have different side effects and problems. Complications from surgery might include infection, nerve damage, and fractures. In addition to the previously noted danger of additional malignancies, radiation therapy can cause skin changes and stiffness in the joints. Despite being typically well tolerated, denosumab may be linked to osteonecrosis of the mandible and hypocalcemia.

GETTING READY FOR THERAPY

To prepare for therapy, a thorough evaluation of the patient's general health must be completed, and each element influencing treatment decisions must be taken into account. Orthopedic surgeons, oncologists, and radiation oncologists may collaborate in a multidisciplinary approach to customize the treatment plan for each patient, and patients who are scheduled for surgery may go through preoperative evaluations to determine their suitability for the procedure.

Cutting-edge treatments like denosumab are combined with more established methods like radiation and surgery to treat giant cell tumors. Making educated decisions requires knowledge of the possible drawbacks and issues connected to each modality. Personalized and interdisciplinary care is necessary to get patients ready for the best possible course of therapy.

4

CHAPTER FOUR

COMPREHENSIVE METHODS FOR TREATING GIANT CELL TUMORS

COMPLEMENTARY AND ALTERNATIVE MEDICINE

Integrative medicine appears as a comprehensive approach in the field of giant cell tumor (GCT) care, addressing the physical, emotional, and spiritual elements of a patient's well-being by combining traditional medical treatments with complementary therapies. Integrative medicine recognizes that treating the patient as a whole, as opposed to just the illness, is important. It entails cooperation between medical specialists from different specialties, such as mental health specialists, alternative medicine practitioners, and traditional medicine doctors.

Integrative medicine can be incorporated into the GCT care paradigm to provide patients with a more thorough and individualized course of therapy. This could entail complementary therapies including acupuncture, massage therapy, and herbal medicine in addition to surgery, chemotherapy, and radiation therapy. Integrative medicine seeks to improve the quality of life for patients with giant cell tumors by promoting the body's natural healing processes.

DIET AND WAY OF LIFE

To treat giant cell tumors holistically, diet and lifestyle are crucial. The immune system and the body's capacity to withstand the effects of treatment are both enhanced by a well-balanced diet tailored to the individual's needs. Patients receiving GCT care may benefit from an adequate intake of vital nutrients, including vitamins, minerals, and antioxidants, as this can improve their general health and resilience.

Furthermore, a healthy lifestyle is essential to the holistic method. Frequent exercise supports stress management and enhances mental health in addition to preserving physical strength. Giant cell tumor patients' general health can be improved by making lifestyle changes like quitting smoking and drinking alcohol in moderation. Together with medical interventions, these integrative strategies support a comprehensive and well-rounded approach to GCT care.

PAIN CONTROL

A key component of comprehensive treatment for giant cell tumors is effective pain management. Patients frequently feel pain of varied intensities as a result of the tumor itself and the therapies used to treat the illness. A variety of techniques, such as pharmacological interventions, physical therapy, and alternative therapies, are included in holistic approaches to pain management.

Pharmacological therapies strive to minimize adverse effects while achieving pain relief through the use of analgesic drugs customized to each patient's unique pain profile. To increase mobility and functionality and, consequently, quality of life, physical therapy can be very helpful. Complementary approaches, such as acupuncture and mindfulness-based techniques, are also increasingly integrated into pain management protocols, offering non-pharmacological alternatives to address pain and improve overall well-being.

EMOTIONAL WELL-BEING

Caring for the emotional well-being of individuals with giant cell tumors is an integral aspect of holistic healthcare. A cancer diagnosis, coupled with the challenges of treatment, can evoke a range of emotions, including anxiety, depression, and fear. Holistic approaches recognize the interconnectedness of the mind and body, emphasizing the importance of addressing emotional well-being alongside physical health.

Psychosocial support, including counseling and support groups, provides a forum for patients to vent their worries, exchange experiences, and receive guidance in coping with the emotional impact of GCT. Mind-body activities like as meditation and mindfulness are increasingly incorporated into holistic treatment programs, enhancing emotional resilience and aiding in stress management.

CHAPTER FIVE

PATIENT NARRATIVES AND PERSPECTIVES

EXPERIENCES IN REAL LIFE

Patient viewpoints provide a deep understanding of the daily realities of people coping with a range of medical illnesses. These personal accounts give medical diagnoses a human face while illuminating the daily struggles, victories, and emotional ups and downs that frequently accompany a health journey. Authenticity is resonant with real-life experiences, which capture subtleties that clinical descriptions could miss. Patients become storytellers through these narratives, sharing priceless knowledge that goes beyond medical textbooks.

Every real-life experience is distinct, molded by the interaction of cultural backgrounds, personal situations, and individual resiliency. From the first symptoms and diagnosis to the course of treatment and recovery, these tales frequently illustrate the highs and lows of navigating the healthcare system. They shed light on the significance of providing holistic care by highlighting the psychological and emotional aspects of recovery in addition to the physical. By sharing their stories, sufferers help others develop empathy and lessen stigma by advancing our understanding of sickness as a group.

ADAPTIVE TECHNIQUES

Overcoming the obstacles posed by disease requires the creation of coping mechanisms that differ greatly from person to person. To adjust to new circumstances while maintaining a feeling of identity and agency, patients must engage in a complex dance between vulnerability and resilience. Coping tactics include a wide range of techniques, such as having a positive outlook, asking for emotional support, researching alternative therapies, and practicing self-care.

Patients often verbalize the growth of their coping techniques over time, suggesting a dynamic process of trial and error. Managing the physical symptoms, coping with the prognosis's uncertainty, and adapting to daily routine adjustments may all be part of the process. Beyond the person, coping involves the assistance of close friends and family, medical professionals, and the larger community. Peer support groups, where common experiences provide a sense of understanding and camaraderie, might provide comfort to certain patients.

SUPPORT NETWORKS

The complexes webs of support that help people get through the difficulties of disease are often the central themes of patient stories. These networks include family, friends, caregivers, and even online communities; they go well beyond the confines of the clinical context. It is impossible to exaggerate the importance of support networks since they stand as pillars of strength when people are most vulnerable.

In addition to providing practical assistance with everyday tasks, emotional support, and advocacy within the healthcare system, family and friends frequently play a critical role. Additionally, caregivers make a huge contribution by skillfully and compassionately negotiating the complications of caregiving. Online communities give patients in the digital age a way to connect with people going through similar things, which helps them feel understood and like they belong.

Healthcare providers are an essential component of the support system in a larger sense, helping patients by explaining treatment options, providing comfort, and answering worries. When these different tiers of care work together, they form a safety net that gives patients the resilience and heightened feeling of community they need to face health issues.

CHAPTER SIX

GETTING AROUND THE HEALTHCARE SYSTEM

PUTTING TOGETHER A MEDICAL TEAM

In the complicated terrain of the healthcare system, having a competent and collaborative healthcare team is vital for effective and thorough patient care. A range of experts, including primary care physicians, specialists, nurses, pharmacists, and other allied health workers, usually make up a healthcare team. Every team member has a distinct responsibility when it comes to treating various facets of a patient's health. Building a solid rapport and open lines of communication with these specialists guarantees that patients receive individualized, well-coordinated care.

Patients should actively choose their healthcare team, taking into account qualities like communication style, experience, and level of knowledge. To ensure that all facets of the patient's health are taken care of and to facilitate communication between various experts, the primary care physician frequently acts as the central coordinator. More emphasis is being placed on shared and collaborative decision-making models, which empower patients to actively participate with their medical team in formulating well-informed treatment regimens.

SPEAKING WITH MEDICAL PROFESSIONALS

A key component of high-quality healthcare is efficient patient-provider communication. Patients can actively participate in their care when there is open and honest communication between them and their caregivers. When speaking with medical professionals about their symptoms, worries, and preferred course of treatment, patients should feel at ease. Healthcare providers should, in turn, communicate diagnoses, available treatments, and likely results in a clear and intelligible manner.

In addition to writing down any questions or concerns they may have, patients are advised to bring a friend or family member to the meeting to offer support and help in understanding the information being given. Additionally, by enabling secure messaging with healthcare practitioners and simple access to medical information, the use of technology—such as patient portals and electronic health records—can improve communication.

SECOND THOUGHTS AND LOBBYING

Getting a second opinion is a smart move when navigating the healthcare system, particularly when dealing with serious or complex medical issues. Obtaining a second opinion can yield more information, validate diagnoses, and suggest different courses of action. It is important for patients to feel comfortable approaching their primary care physician or specialist about getting a second opinion, and most medical professionals value and encourage this proactive approach to making healthcare decisions.

Another essential component of navigating the healthcare system is patient advocacy. To guarantee that their rights are upheld, their concerns are acknowledged, and their preferences are taken into account during the decision-making process, patients or their appointed advocates are essential. Clearly expressing one's choices, being aware of available treatments, and obtaining informed consent are some examples of advocacy. Patient advocacy can be particularly important when dealing with complex treatment regimens, negotiating insurance challenges, and managing end-of-life care decisions.

INSURANCE AND FINANCIAL ISSUES

Dealing with insurance and financial issues is a common part of navigating the healthcare system. It's critical to comprehend health insurance terms, such as deductibles, co-pays, and networks, to make wise judgments regarding the use of healthcare resources. When in doubt, patients should contact their insurance companies to get more information. Patients should also take the initiative to confirm that certain procedures, drugs, and medical professionals are covered.

Patients may experience a great deal of stress due to financial issues, therefore it's critical to discuss these worries honestly with medical providers. Open communication about financial concerns can help healthcare professionals tailor their recommendations to align with the patient's financial situation, ensuring that the proposed treatment plans are realistic and feasible. Financial counselors are available at many healthcare facilities to offer guidance on navigating the financial aspects of medical care, including assistance with insurance claims, financial assistance programs, and payment plans.

CHAPTER SEVEN

AFTER TREATMENT LIFE

RECUPERATION AND REHABILITATION

Following treatment is a critical stage in the cancer patient's journey, at which time they begin the process of recuperation and rehabilitation. In an attempt to restore a sense of normalcy, survivors must consider social, emotional, and physical factors. A gradual return to regular activities that are adapted to the requirements and capabilities of the individual is common in physical rehabilitation. Exercises that increase strength, flexibility, and endurance may be a part of this, supporting the restoration of general physical health.

Survivors may have emotional difficulties transitioning to life after treatment and managing the psychological effects of their cancer experience. The importance of therapy interventions, counseling, and support groups is crucial in overcoming emotional obstacles and building resilience. Rebuilding relationships and reestablishing contact with a support system are the main goals of social rehabilitation, which helps survivors work through the challenges of reintegrating into their communities.

FOLLOW-UP CARE

Focusing on routine medical check-ups and evaluations to track the patient's health state, follow-up care is an essential part of life after treatment. These consultations are intended to identify any possible recurrence or persistent adverse effects as soon as possible. Follow-up care regimens, which combine physical examinations, imaging tests, and bloodwork, are frequently customized to the particular cancer type and treatment received.

Over time, the number of follow-up visits may drop, but continuous monitoring is still crucial. In addition to addressing physical health, these check-ups give survivors a chance to talk about any new worries or emotional difficulties. In the post-treatment phase, the cooperative interaction between survivors and healthcare providers encourages a proactive approach to preserving general well-being.

LONG-TERM MONITORING AND SURVIVORSHIP

Going beyond standard follow-up care, long-term monitoring is a crucial part of survivorship. It includes the overall health and wellness of those who have finished their initial course of cancer therapy. When it comes to the aftereffects of cancer and its therapies, survivors frequently encounter particular difficulties. These can include possible long-term negative effects on their physical and mental health as well as their quality of life.

Long-term survivability requires a multifaceted approach that includes lifestyle adjustments, continuous emotional support, and knowledge of possible aftereffects. Proactive management of survivorship difficulties involves regular monitoring for complications associated with late treatment and screening for subsequent malignancies. The area of survivorship care is growing and now acknowledges the value of survivorship care plans, which provide individualized support to help patients adjust to life following treatment.

HANDLING RECURRENCE FEAR

For many cancer survivors, fear of recurrence is a frequent and natural concern. To overcome this fear, one must recognize and comprehend how it affects one's mental health. Giving survivors information on the chance of recurrence according to their particular cancer kind, stage, and course of therapy might help them understand and control their fears.

Psychosocial support, such as therapy and support groups, gives survivors a forum to talk about their fears and coping mechanisms. Creating a customized strategy for handling recurrence anxiety may entail lifestyle modifications, mindfulness practices, and continuing consultation with medical professionals. Adopting a proactive approach and concentrating on controllable parts of life can enable survivors to manage the emotional side of life after treatment and improve their overall resilience.